SLEEP SOUNDLY

Fall Asleep In Five Easy Steps

By: Dr. James Kohan

Speedy Publishing LLC

2658 Del Mar Hts Rd, #358

Del Mar, CA 92014

www.SleepDisordersInformation.org

DISCLAIMER

This book is not intended as medical advice. It is also not intended to prevent, diagnose, treat or cure disease. Instead the book is intended only to share the unofficial research and opinion of the author. The information is provided for educational purposes only, not as treatment instructions for any disease or ailment. Much of the book is a statement of opinion in areas where the facts are controversial or do not exist. The information in this book should not be considered any more valid than any other type of informal opinion.

The information was not written to replace the advice or care of a qualified health care professional. Be sure to check with your own qualified health care provider before beginning any protocols or procedures discussed in this book, or before stopping or altering any diet, lifestyle, or other therapies previously recommended to you by your health care provider.

The treatments described in this book may have side effects and carry other known and unknown risks and health hazards. The statements in this book have not been evaluated by the United States FDA. Use of the information in this book is at your own risk.

This book is dedicated to all the sleepless who suffer in silence.

"Sleep is the best meditation."

—Dalai Lama

A MESSAGE TO ALL SLEEPLESS SOULS

Sleeping is one of life's simplest and most relaxing pleasures. I say pleasure because, in all honesty, that's what it truly is. When we sleep, our body benefits from it the most. I am Dr. James Kohan and for the better part of three decades, I have been studying sleep and all its aspects —more so to help those who are in dire need of it. In years of study and working with patients I've found two critical benefits to sleep:

Dreaming. When your body enters a relaxed state and you slowly drift into unconsciousness, you get to experience what is usually known as R.E.M. This phase in sleep allows you to dream. While dreaming might seem mundane, in reality, it's what keeps you thinking, learning and remembering more fully. It allows you to experience life more fully through your sense and emotion, as well as to concentrate and direct your attention. Without dreaming, the brain would never be able to deal with all the stimulation that it receives each and every second of the waking day.

Rejuvenation. Sleep offers our bodies sanctuary from all the waking activities we perform. Like it or not, the body is like a machine —subject to wear and tear— and if not taken cared of properly, would deteriorate and diminish in performance before its supposed time. A good amount of quality sleep keeps you going every single day.

If you find yourself with difficulties in falling asleep or staying asleep, or are cranky, moody, slow on the uptake and generally lack an ability to go about daily activities, then relax —you are in the right place. After thousands of patients, I understand —you are NOT to blame! You are simply exhausted —physically & mentally.

I've dedicated my life's learning and medical practice to helping people with sleep problems. If you are anxious for answers right away, download The ABZZZ's of Sleep: Insomnia, Sleep Apnea & Other Sleeping Disorders as my gift to you (retails for $9.99):

http://SleepDisordersInformation.org/sign-up

Here's a chance to reclaim what is rightfully yours… your rest, rejuvenation and relaxation! Loss of sleep and/or the inability to have any (consistent quality sleep) can be more detrimental to your health than you might be willing to recognize. I earnestly hope that by reading this book, you will find yourself in the arms of restful slumber once more. For all your inquiries on sleep disorders, I'm here to help. Feel free to send me an email.

All the best,
Dr. James Kohan
dr.jameskohan@sleepdisordersinformation.org

Table of Contents

INTRODUCTION

Over the 30 years that I've spent helping patients with various sleep disorders, I have come to understand that education, combined with proper information, is the most effective tool when it comes to helping someone with a sleep problem. Here, in this book, one of my goals was to introduce the basics of sleep to allow an understanding of both the normal process and the variations which result in problems related to it.

A sleep problem can develop and progress in a very subtle way. Symptoms can be the result of many different underlying causes. Likewise, treatment can also be a chronic ongoing process with individualized variations in standard treatment. The patient has to be actively involved in the process and this is best achieved by having the "whole program bought into." In other words, the patient has to be taught how to monitor and adapt their own sleep-wake schedule, much like a diabetic patient needs to learn how to monitor finger-stick glucose values and adjust their diet.

In this short overview book of sleep in health and disease, it is my earnest hope that the reader may come to appreciate the full picture of how and why we sleep, come to terms with what can go wrong and how to approach sleep disorders with the proper knowledge and understanding of how to address them.

CHAPTER 1 – SLEEP BASICS

Sleep is like breathing. You don't think about it much until you can't do it. You know that you need both, but you may not understand all the details of exactly why you need them or what they do for your body. It may be that you only try to learn the details when you experience some form of insomnia. If you want to combat insomnia and get back to a regular sleep pattern, you first have to learn some of the sleep basics.

Sleep Stages

Stage 1: The first of the four stages of sleep is a "transition" stage from a waking state to true sleep. It only lasts a few minutes at most in the beginning of the night. Even though it is a transition towards true sleep, there is no consciousness. If you are awakened during this stage, you may THINK that you were awake, but you would have NO MEMORY or what just occurred.

Stage 2: The 2nd stage of sleep is called "light" sleep. It is called the first stage of "true sleep," as there are specific telltale brain wave patterns called "sleep spindles" and "K complexes" which distinguish this stage. It is the most common stage of sleep, especially as we age into adulthood and old age.

Stages 3: Stage 3 is called "deep" sleep. This stage is characterized by "Delta" or slow brain waves. There used to be a further division into stage 3 and 4 based on the percentage of these Delta waves, but this is no longer done. This is the time during which all of your body systems get the most rest. They are functioning at minimal levels. Because of this low level of functioning, your senses are not as in tune with the environment as they are when you are awake. Because this is when you are least responsive to the environment, it is most difficult to be awakened from Stage 3 sleep.

Stage 4: Stage 4 is called "Rapid Eye Movement" sleep or REM. This is the "dream" sleep stage. There is a general disconnect of the brain from the monitoring of body functions, as the brain is in the realm of dreams.

One obvious occurrence is that we are paralyzed during REM, so the body does not act out the brain's dreams. The brain also does not regulate breathing, heart rate or body temperature during this stage. This is why when you awaken during the night feeling cold or warm; it is usually at a time when you are dreaming.

We go through all stages of sleep in a revolving cycle which lasts 60-90 minutes throughout the night. Typically, you will cycle 4 to 6 times each night. Stage 3 ("deep" sleep) occurs mostly in the first half of the night, while REM occurs for longer periods of time as the night progresses. The longest REM or "dream" cycle occurs just before you wake up in the morning. This is usually the reason why you have more trouble becoming alert (waking up) if you have to force yourself up 30 minutes earlier in the morning. As mentioned above, the most common stage of sleep for an adult is stage 2 ("light" sleep), but up until age 20 it is stage 3 ("deep" sleep). Somewhere between age 20 and 30, the % of "deep" sleep decreases and the % of "light" sleep increases. At around this age, the amount of REM ("Dream" sleep) stabilizes at 20%, where it remains for the rest of adulthood.

The Purpose of Sleep

The purpose of sleep is best understood as a time for regeneration and renewal. In simple terms, the body's muscles and organs are regenerated during "non-REM" sleep, especially stage 3 or "Deep" sleep, while the brain is "renewed" during REM sleep. It is during "deep" sleep wherein the human growth hormone is secreted by the brain, stimulating the body's restoration. During the dream stage, it's as if the brain's "tapes" (the day's events and our emotional response to them) are replayed and erased to allow better concentration and mental capacity for the next day.

The Sleep-Wake Brain System

Sleep is governed by its own brain system, as is wakefulness. They each take their turn at being the most prominent during certain times of the day. This is the so-called Circadian Rhythm system which is our "internal clock". It is housed inside the brain in the Pineal gland. It is what causes us to feel alert during the day, and sleepy during the night, regardless of the amount of sleep or work that you do and whether you watch the clock on the wall. It is a natural system, but it too can be fooled by bad (or even well-intended) habits, medical conditions or medications.

CHAPTER 2 – WHAT IS INSOMNIA

If you have ever felt that your insomnia was a bit more than just a "restless night" experienced by people who normally sleep well, you were correct. People who experience insomnia can toss and turn for hours on a regular basis before they actually fall asleep. When they do fall asleep, they don't sleep as deeply as other people and as a result are more prone to waking up at various times throughout the night. Unlike the average person who might wake up through the night for short periods of time without even realizing it, the person who has insomnia will be alert and awake for long periods of time. One of the reasons this may happen is that people who have insomnia are also people with a lot of physical tension. You may have mentioned this and been dismissed, but the proof is in the fact that people who have insomnia demonstrate a higher heart rate and more muscle tension than the average sleeper.

When you have a day of hard physical labor, you may notice that you sleep better at night. This is because most people experience body temperatures that fluctuate from high to low throughout the day, while some insomniacs only experience a very mild version of this fluctuation, part of which can occur due to physical activity. This natural lack of fluctuation means that your body is in the same state when you lay down to sleep as it was in the middle of the day. To make matters worse, the lack of sleep may cause a lack of energy through the day so it can be difficult to change this cycle.

Based on numerous studies to date, it would seem that the cause and effect of insomnia are somewhat reversed as to how they are labeled. It would seem that the body systems that balance the wake and sleep systems are out of balance themselves so that when you should feel awake, you are tired, but when you should feel tired, you feel wide awake. Further, when you are tossing and turning at night and you blame your thoughts for keeping you awake, those thoughts are not to blame. They are simply the result of lying awake with nothing to do but think.

The good news is that it is possible to use techniques that can balance the systems. Once you learn to make your sleep system stronger and take steps to prepare for a good night's sleep, the body will respond with increasing amounts of restful nights. You may have tried some techniques of your own in an attempt to get a good night's sleep.

Do you plan to get to bed sooner in the hopes that you will get more sleep? Perhaps you try to give yourself a means to relax in bed, like watching a late show or reading a book. Are you self-medicating to try to physically force yourself to sleep? Have you noticed a decrease in your activity during the day as a result of your sleepless nights?

It could be that your focus on trying to get a good night's sleep has actually forced your body to change from an occasional bout with insomnia to an ongoing issue. The more you focus on the insomnia itself, the more prevalent it is. To change the course of events, you will need to learn to change the thought process and behaviors that cause them.

People who experience insomnia as well as health professionals who treat it may be wasting time when treating it as a psychiatric ailment. It is sometimes simplistic to think that insomnia is causing a psychological condition, like anxiety or depression. It is common for an insomniac, and even the physician or therapist, to think that the insomnia is the "cause". While insomnia or even any bad night of sleep can worsen feelings of anxiety and depression, unrecognized depression is frequently the cause of chronic insomnia. Making the diagnosis, correcting the bad habits which propagate poor sleep and initiating a plan to treat depression frequently takes a cooperative approach between the insomniac and his/her medical professional.

Chapter 3 – Step 1: Change How You Think About Sleep

Of all the things that you blame your insomnia on, negative thinking should be at the top of your list.

After reading that first statement you probably thought something like "Yes, those racing thoughts do keep me up at night," which is not what was meant. Those racing thoughts you have at night are not the cause of your insomnia; they are a direct result of your insomnia. The thoughts that came before your head ever hit the pillow are the ones that are causing the insomnia.

If your thoughts are powerful enough to cause insomnia, that would also mean they are powerful enough to reverse it. Once you accept that fact, you won't just be able to end your insomnia; you will be able to change an entire range of things in your life just by changing the way you think about them. This is called cognitive restructuring and it works with just about anything you do in life.

Once you realize the power that your very thoughts have over something as complex as your sleep patterns, you will begin applying those techniques to other areas of your life and experience an increase in self-confidence as well as energy. Negative thoughts will begin to lose their sway over you.

Consider the Placebo Effect

Are you still having trouble convincing yourself that thoughts can change your sleep patterns? Consider the placebo effect. About 1/3 of patients who are given a placebo while participating in medical studies experience the exact same level of relief as the patients who are given the actual medications. This extends to even the most powerful of drugs, such as morphine.

Stress and Wakefulness

You may tend to blame your lack of sleep due to the stress in your life. This act alone can actually lead to a lack of sleep. Negative Sleep Thoughts (NSTs) occur, when you basically build the foundation for a sleepless night before you ever get to bed. Essentially, you talk about sleep in such a negative way that by the end of the night you have already convinced yourself that you are not going to sleep well. By the time you go to bed, you keep yourself awake with these thoughts. Do any of the statements below sound familiar?

Negative Sleep Thoughts You Should Do Away With
• "I know I'm going to toss and turn all night."
• "I never get a good night's sleep."
• "This insomnia is draining all my energy."

When you talk like this or even think like this, you put your body in a state of stress. This stress can cause you to experience an inability to fall asleep since a stressed body is fully alert and in fight or flight mode.

If you don't believe this, think about the last time you had a tooth pulled. You were terrified and gripping the chair. The dentist repeatedly told you to calm down or the numbing medicine could not work. You may have even had to get an extra shot. This is not due to your body's natural responses, but to the stress that you put on the body as a result of your negative thoughts.

CHAPTER 4 – STEP 2: TAKE CONTROL OF YOUR LIFE & SLEEP

The way you manage your life during the day has an impact on your sleep patterns long before you say "good night". In this section of the report you will see how environmental factors and the way you respond to them can determine the way you sleep at night. You will also learn some direct methods you can use in order to create the perfect environment for a good night's sleep.

Increase Your Energy

A minimum of twenty-ie25% of adult Americans are overweight and inactive. The trickle effect can be seen in the increasing numbers of overweight children. The body was not meant to live such a lifestyle and the impact can be seen in the increasing amounts of people who suffer from heart disease, diabetes, high blood pressure, depression and some cancers. Ten percent (10%) of the deaths that occur in the United States are caused by inactivity. Ironically, the people who suffer from depression also suffer from a low self-esteem that can be greatly improved with increased activity. A reduction in anxiety, stress, pain, and disability can also occur with increased activity while improvements can be seen in mood, energy, body image, health and quality of life.

For maximum benefits, exercise should be done 3to 6 hours before going to bed. This gives the body time to cool down and "unwind" before sleep. The physical stress placed on the body will naturally induce a deeper sleep as the body tries to compensate for the physical stressor, which is wholly different from a mental stressor. The body also responds to the night and day cycle, so people who exercise outside will see even more benefits to their sleep schedule as the body responds to the natural cycle induced by melatonin, the hormone that regulates sleep.

When your eyes are exposed to sunlight, the melatonin levels decrease and the body temperature rises in an expression of wakefulness. On the other hand, when the eyes no longer see sunlight, the body responds by increasing melatonin and decreasing the body temperature in preparation for sleep.

Without this exposure to sunlight, the natural sleep cycle of the body is disrupted. For example, ninety percent (90%) of blind people experience sleeping problems due to the need for exposure to light and dark through the eyes. People who do not expose themselves to sunlight may also experience decreased energy and alertness levels as the body is never truly prompted into wakefulness.

Basically, when you expose yourself to sunlight, even if you don't start off by exercising in the sunlight, you are still tuning in your body's natural cycle. Since sleep-onset insomnia is caused in part by the delayed fall of the body temperature, an exposure to sunlight during the early morning hours can cause a decrease in the frequency of the sleep-onset insomnia.

Conversely, people who do not experience sleep-onset insomnia but, instead, experience insomnia in the form of early morning awakenings can benefit from sunlight in the evening hours. Their body temperature rises too quickly and causes them to wake up early. The exposure to bright light during the evening hours can delay this rise in temperature and allow for the continuation of sleep in up to the mid morning hours.

For those who experience a sluggish feeling during the day caused by the insomnia from the night before, breaks during the day experienced in the sunlight can be beneficial when it comes to increasing energy. Furthermore, a lack of exposure to sunlight often causes a reduced vitamin D level, which in turn can cause a decrease in energy, as well as numerous other side effects. Because of this, exposure to sunlight and the increase in vitamin D levels can cause an almost immediate feeling of rejuvenation.

CHAPTER 5 – STEP 3: REDUCE YOUR STRESS

Have you ever compared yourself to other people who experience similar life situations and wondered how they seem, to not only manage their stress so easily, but also stay healthy and sleep well? The reason is that they have developed a thought process and belief system (whether consciously or unconsciously) that naturally reduces stress levels, even if the environment would seem to increase them.

Keep the Glass Half Full

The optimist sees the glass as half full rather than half empty. They expect positive results and see everything else as a path to even better things. They find the good in any given situation. Losing a job means more time to pursue an even better job. They still experience negative thoughts from time to time, but their mental filter causes them to discard these thoughts and revert to positive ones. Because of this, they experience elevated moods, high levels of energy, and a healthier sense of well-being in general.

Life events can certainly influence the way that you think if you let them. The key is to take back control in order to promote positive thoughts, beliefs, and attitudes. Below are some helpful strategies to that end.

Positive Attitude Reinforcement Tips

- A setback is a detour, not a dead end. The end of a relationship does not mean the end of all relationships. Not getting approved for a loan today does not mean not getting approved for a loan forever.

- One issue does not make a lifetime of failure. Words like "ever" and "always" only apply to fairy tales. If you don't get hired after one interview, it does not mean you will never get a job.

- Embrace positive events. When you focus on positive events, they happen more frequently. Assume that one positive event is the beginning of a pattern rather than a fluke. After all, you assumed that about negative events and got exactly what you expected.

- Accept your lack of control. The only one you have control of is yourself. You are not responsible for how the environment responds to you, but you are responsible for how you respond to it.

- Make use of a positive mantra. Repetition is the key to belief. As a child you learned the alphabet by repeating it so many times that you couldn't forget it now if you tried. Create a mantra and repeat it to yourself as needed. For instance, repeat "I am worthy of success" throughout the day.

- Be thankful. Every day you wake up with something to be thankful for. The fact that you can get out of bed is positive. The fact that you have the mental ability to think is reason enough to be thankful.

- Develop an allergy to pessimism. Attitudes are contagious. Make sure you are around positive people.

As a result of your efforts, you will experience fewer negative thoughts and emotions even if your environment does or does not change.

Laughter is Still the Best Medicine

Laughter produces serotonin, as well as endorphins that can induce a state of euphoria and numb pain. It can even boost the immune system. Humor is one of the most effective combatants to stress. It reduces anxiety and anger while also allowing for a change in perspective. Humor allows you to see the humanity in your faults. All those people you think are laughing at your faults? They have their own and will be stunned to see how effectively you embrace yours. Your humor will increase your self-esteem level. At the same time, the mirror effect you see in other people as they respond to you will also help enhance your self-esteem.

CHAPTER 6 – STOP RELYING ON MEDICATIONS

Sleeping pills were once a popular method by which insomnia was treated. Note: the method was popular, but not effective. Like many other medications on the market today, sleeping pills treated some of the symptoms without ever getting to the cause of insomnia. When you don't treat the cause, the symptoms only increase. When the symptoms increase, so does the dosage; when the dosage increases, so does the tolerance and dependence. And round and round she goes, it's a vicious cycle. Many people take these pills under the illusion that they will somehow regain control of the sleeping portion of their life. Instead, they lose control to the pharmacy. Like any other medication, these pills were never meant to be a long term solution, but should have been a short term one to treat the symptoms until the cause was found and treated.

Sleeping pills can be beneficial if they are only used occasionally. If a significant event such as a death or some event that causes short term stress is experienced, sleeping pills can help you sleep as you learn to cope with the event in a healthy way.

To prevent creating a situation of long term insomnia while taking sleeping pills, take them under the following conditions:

When To Use Sleeping Pills

- Use the medication in combination with the techniques found in this book. As the techniques are used more and more and are effective, decrease the frequency of taking medications.

- Use the smallest dose possible.

- Never use the pills two days in a row or before experiencing 2 or more sleepless nights. This will decrease the risk of dependency as well as ensure that you practice non-medicinal techniques.

- Do not exceed the prescribed dosage and only use pills with a short half-life.

Stop the Use of Pills

Cut your dose in half one night out of your schedule. Do this on a schedule until you are sleeping well through the night while only using half a dose. It is best to choose a night that follows an active day but not precede a stressful one. Repeat this process until you are only taking half a dose every night that you use sleeping pills. Repeat the process by eliminating the dose altogether in the same fashion. For instance, if you originally cut your dose in half once every two weeks, do the same for eliminating the dose. If you use more than one type of sleeping pill, repeat this process for each type, one at a time. For instance, do not cut the dose in half for any two medications at once. Keep in mind that procrastination only increases anxiety, so the sooner you take these steps, the easier they will be to complete.

CHAPTER 7 – RE-CREATE A SLEEP CYCLE

Everyone has little habits they have to do at certain times. Though some of these habits are bad, others can be manipulated to induce a response from your body. For instance, some people like to have a cigarette after eating, otherwise they'd have an anxiety.

Though, the aforementioned instance is not a favorable habit, the idea is to use that same system to create a new sleep cycle.

Creating a Sleep Cycle

1. Create a bedtime ritual. Your body needs to go through a series of events on a regular basis in order to develop a pattern that is done without thought. Most people get up and brush their teeth every morning along with other morning rituals, but if they were to actually try to remember whether or not they brushed their teeth, they may not remember the actual event. Create this same atmosphere using at least four steps that are repeated before you go to bed each night. This prepares your body for the next step of sleeping. Below are some suggestions:

   • Tidy the kitchen.

   • Get the coffee pot ready for morning.

   • Lock the doors.

   • Complete your hygiene ritual.

2. Force your body to associate the bedroom with sleep. This is not a place for television or computer, but for sleep.

3. Take action after 30 minutes. If you are not asleep within 30 minutes, use the exercises below to help reduce your anxiety and get to sleep.

    • First exercise: Go to another room, turn on a light and do something simple that requires little thought.

    • Second exercise: Sitting on the edge of your bed with your hands relaxed by your sides, head tilted forward towards your chest, and your shoulders stooped, breathe in through your nose and hold it for five seconds. Let your breath out. As you breathe in, visualize the air filling your lungs and body and then visualize it leaving your body in the same detail. Do this for a few moments or until you are sleepy.

4. Keep on a waking schedule. Set your alarm for the same time every day. Your body is searching for a sleeping pattern and will gladly embrace a waking schedule. Soon you will wake up without an alarm at the same time every day, which will in turn help you fall asleep at the same time every night.

5. Turn the clock away from you. It does nothing to help you fall asleep when you continuously keep looking at it. Turn it away from the bed if need be.

6. Stop worrying about sleep. If you are not getting enough sleep, thinking about it will not make it happen. Let the natural chain of events unfold so that you are in a positive frame of mind, free from

worry. With that being said, assume that the steps above will help you even if it takes a bit of time and practice.

CHAPTER 8 – SHARING THE BED

If you are a sensitive sleeper, sharing the bed with someone may not present the ideal situation for you. Movements or sounds that your bed partner makes can cause you to wake up frequently through the night. Not only is this going to make you to feel tired the next day; it is not going to do anything to promote positive relations with your partner. You may even start to feel resentment. Below are some ways you can share the bed and still get a good night's sleep.

Accommodate Boundary Issues

Some people like to feel the touch of someone next to them all night long. Others require their own separate space to get comfortable. The most obvious thing that has to be done in order to ensure that you both get a good night's rest is to discuss the issue and stress the fact that your physical contact limitations during sleep have nothing to do with a lack of affection. Rather, boundaries need to be set in order to ensure an ongoing affection in the relationship under terms that do not negatively impact the sleep schedule.

Bed Sharing Terms & Agreement
1. You can share a space without sharing a bed. Instead of sleeping in one large bed, push two smaller beds together so that you are sharing a space, but your body can recognize the difference between the beds and respond accordingly. You won't feel your partner move in their bed, but you will be able to be affectionate when the time is right.

2. Use your own blanket. If each partner has their own blanket, the evening will not be spent trying to make one blanket cover two people adequately. You can even keep one large blanket over the two so that the bed does not look odd, but you each have your own cover for the night.

3. Use a quality, firm mattress. A springy mattress responds to every move. A firm mattress does not move as much. Hence, if you do share one mattress with your partner, you won't wake up every time he or she rolls over in the night.

4. Establish a time for affection. Let your partner know that you want to be affectionate. Suggest that you are affectionate before you try to go to sleep, but not during the time you want to sleep. Make your partner feel appreciated, not as if they are being avoided and you will get a guilt free night's sleep. This can even be a part of your "before sleep ritual" and serve as a cue for your body that it is almost time for sleep.

5. Allow room for movement. If you already have a hard time getting to sleep or staying asleep, you don't need any more obstructions to wake you up at night. This includes a wall. If possible, do not push your bed against the wall. If it is against the wall, do not be the one to sleep next to it. A light sleeper can wake up just because his or her hand brushed the wall as they rolled over. This is one obstacle that you can easily eliminate.

6. Use the same schedule. You and your partner should go to bed at the same time. This not only reinforces your bedtime ritual as you and your partner each go through the motions of getting ready for bed. This also eliminates the possibility of your partner waking you up when they come to bed later than you. Another added benefit is that your

affection time will never be compromised.

Chapter 9 – Multiple Lights at The End of The Tunnel

As you might imagine, many of the techniques offered in this report can help with several areas of life other than just sleep. To that end, you can follow a specific schedule to start your journey towards a future of restful nights and stress free days. As you move through the steps, keep in mind that the only way to solve a problem is to get to the root of it and that very statement is the reason why medications do not work when they treat symptoms and not the reason for the symptoms.

From the day you start this program, your goal is going to be to live a happier, healthier lifestyle, empowered by your own positive thoughts. Right now, pick a day on the calendar to start your 30 days of retraining your body and mind to be empowered through positive thinking. Commit to that day.

On the first day as well as the days that follow, you will wake up and be thankful for the day you are going to have. You will be excited about all that you have to look forward to and even the smallest steps that you can take toward your goals. As your feet hit the floor, you will not think about how you slept the night before. Rather, you will embrace the day as it comes, beginning with an affirmation of how worthy you are and how wonderful your day is going to be.

Before you begin any tasks for the day, step out into the sunshine. If you are normally inactive, even those few steps are progress. Recognize it and embrace it. Tomorrow or later in the day, you will take even just a few more steps. You will compare yourself to anyone but yourself and you will recognize this progress as it flows.

Complete your tasks for the day with gratitude in your ability to complete them. When you are with other people, ask yourself how you feel with them. If your mood or energy level is diminished by their presence, simply walk away, seeking bright light or sunshine if possible. When you speak, ask yourself if you are saying anything helpful or if you are adding to negative thoughts. Focus on positive thoughts and words.

Follow through with your bedtime ritual every night. Get up with the alarm every morning and repeat the process. Within a matter of days, possibly even on the first one, you will feel more alert but calmer than you previously were. As the days go on, this feeling will continue to grow.

In the future, if you have trouble sleeping, just refer back to the steps offered in this program. Remember how they helped you sleep better. Repeat them. This will get easier as time goes on and soon enough, the steps will be second nature to you.

Fair warning: Through this process you may find that there are people in your life who leave you feeling drained or who question your new outlook with something akin to hostility. Remember that you have control over yourself and no one else has control over you unless you let them. To that end you may find that you will begin to avoid these people unless you stay around them out of habit. This can be difficult if you are normally a passive person who fears feeling alone. Just remember that your positive attitude is as contagious as a negative one and will actually draw positive people to you.

CHAPTER 10 – RELAXATION ACTIVITY

Self-induced relaxation techniques work best when you can use all of your senses to induce relaxation. Visualize the descriptions as they happen. If possible, sit in a calm, quiet environment with very limited possibility of interruption. Soft, calming music or natural sounds as well as incense may be of benefit. Loose fitting clothes are recommended. Read the method below and memorize it, or record it on an audio device for you to use until you have your technique firmly in place.

Close your eyes and clear your mind. Focus on the act of breathing in the calm cool air and breathing out the tensions from the day. Continue to focus on steady breaths throughout this activity.

Focus on your toes. Imagine relaxation moving over your toes as a warm breeze or warm water. This wave of relaxation moves through your toes, into your feet, and up your calves. Visualize this calming wave as it moves from your toes all the way up to your thighs and through your stomach, chest, and back. You feel your muscles relax as the tension is washed away.

As the tension leaves your feet, legs, chest, stomach and back, the wave of relaxation moves to your fingertips. Feel the warm waves as they move up your hands, arms, and shoulders. It rolls over your neck, jaw, cheeks, forehead, and eyes. Focus on your breathing, notice how calm and regular it is. If thoughts wander into your mind, simply return your focus to your breathing.

Step by step, imagine every part of your body heavy with relief. Aloud, say the words "My arms are heavy." Repeat this phrase three times, each time visualizing and feeling your arms getting a bit heavier. Now, say "My legs are heavy" three times, each time visualizing and feeling your legs get heavier.

Now, your body is getting warm. Say aloud "My arms are warm" three times and imagine the feeling of warmth. Now say, "My legs are heavy" three times and imagine the feeling of warmth. You now feel relaxed and warm. Take a slow deep breath and open your eyes.

RECOMMENDED READING

In over three decades of studying sleep —its purpose, mechanics and how to help those who are in need of it, I have gathered, read and researched upon lots of content that would help me enlighten and broaden my knowledge and understanding. Below are some of the materials that have enriched my learning further. I earnestly hope these books will do the same for you. You can check them out on my site here:

http://SleepDisordersInformation.org/recommended

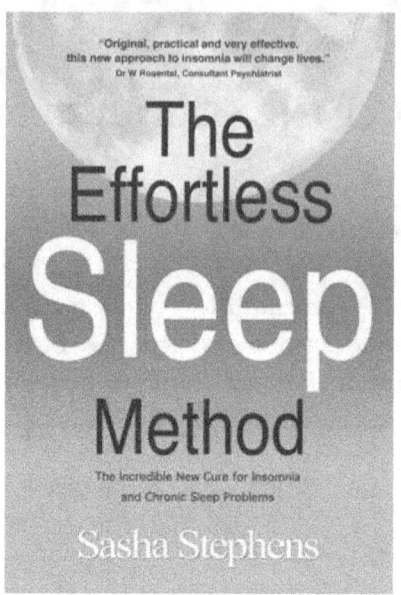

The Effortless Sleep Method: The Incredible New Cure for Insomnia and Chronic Sleep Problems

This book is what every insomniac needs. With very original, practical and effective sleep tips guaranteed to give you an effortless sleep.

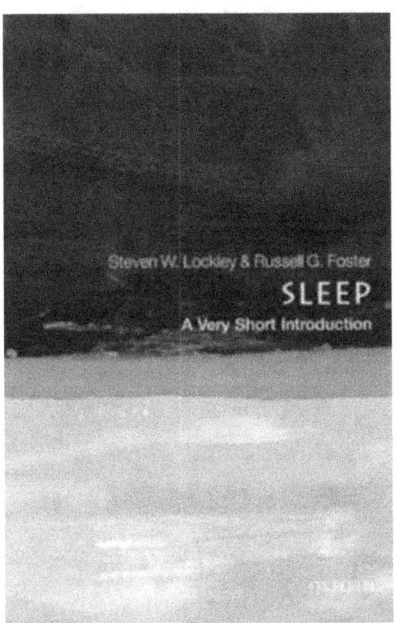

Sleep: A Very Short Introduction

We spend almost around a third of our lives asleep. When know that it's vital to our health and bodily functions. But just how much sleep is actually considered "healthy"? This book will provide answers to a whole lot of sleep related questions.

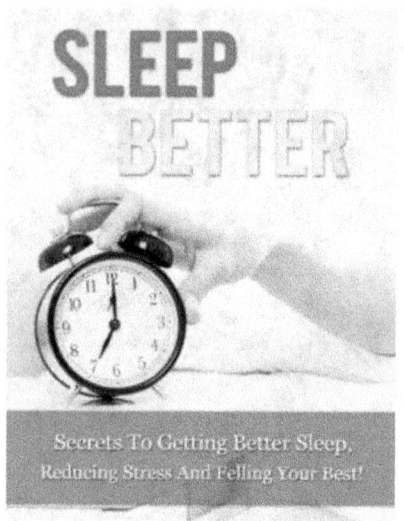

S

leep Better: Secrets To Getting Better Sleep, Reducing Stress, And Feeling Your Best! (Sleep Better, sleeping disorders)

Reach your goal towards getting better sleep quality with methodical strategies and tested steps. Reduce your stress and feel your best each and every single time you wake up.

THE SURPRISING SCIENCE OF
THE MIND AT REST

the   secret

world

of   sleep

PENELOPE A. LEWIS

The Secret World of Sleep: The Surprising Science of the Mind at Rest (MacSci)

This book provides the latest research on sleep, resting and how to get more of both by laying simple truth and information. Authored by an authority in the field of sleep, Lewis fills in the gaps to uncovering and learning the secret world of sleep.

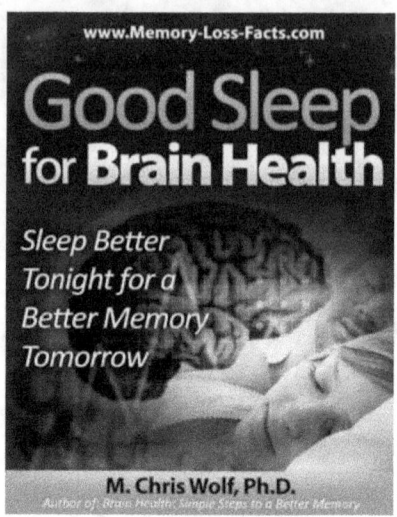

Good Sleep for Brain Health: Sleep Better Tonight for a Better Memory Tomorrow

A healthy brain for a better memory. Get a good night's sleep with the help of this book and improve your body's overall health and at the same time, boost your brain's capacity for memory retention.

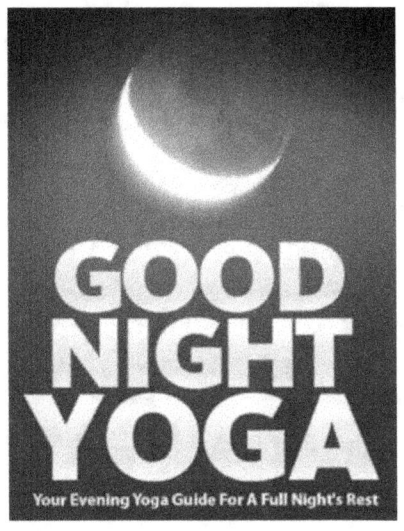

Good Night Yoga: Your Evening Yoga Guide For A Full Night's Rest (Just Do Yoga)

Sleep well to Good Night Yoga. Yes, you heard right! This book holds powerful Yoga relaxation routine and techniques to soothe and calm yourself in preparation for a good night's rest.

ABOUT THE AUTHOR

Dr. Kohan was educated at the University Of Virginia where he also received his M.D. from the School of Medicine. He finished his residency training at Long Island College Hospital in Brooklyn, NYC.

Dr. Kohan completed a fellowship in Pulmonary Medicine at the University of Rochester. He finished sleep medicine training at St. Mary's Sleep Center in Rochester, NY, which at the time was one of only five sleep labs in the U.S.

Dr. Kohan has founded and directed sleep labs throughout the world, including New Hartford, NY; Ljubljana, Slovenia; Honolulu and Hilo, HI: Pago Pago, Am. Samoa; Anchorage, AK; San Diego and El Centro, CA. He has seen the field of sleep medicine grow from a medical curiosity to one of everyday recognition.

You can find Dr. Kohan on Google+ and Facebook.

www.ingramcontent.com/pod-product-compliance
Lightning Source LLC
Chambersburg PA
CBHW070844290526
45795CB00002B/974